Baking Soda Wonder

Baking Soda Home Remedies For Cleaning, Hygiene And Health

(Secrets To Natural Cleaning And Vibrant Health)

MERCY MITCH

ISBN-13:978-1508965985

ISBN-10:1508965986

DEDICATION

To all women who desire a squeaky-clean home.

TABLE OF CONTENT

INTRODUCTION

An Insight Into The Wonders Of Baking Soda

Baking soda is a white powder with an alkaline taste. Also known as sodium bicarbonate, bicarbonate of soda and bicarb, it is readily available as it is found naturally dissolved in mineral springs all over the world.

Baking soda is incredibly versatile and amazingly cheap particularly when purchased in bulk. Originally meant for cooking, it has proven to be highly useful in various ways, including cleaning and medical purposes.

When used in cooking, baking soda acts as a leavening agent that causes baked goods to rise. Once it is added to the batter, it reacts with an acidic ingredient in the recipe such as honey, lemon juice, milk or brown sugar. This reaction creates carbon dioxide that expands the dough and as it bakes, it rises. It is used in baking breads, cakes and cookies.

As a cleaning agent, it is safe and contains no toxic substances that could be detrimental to health - both of humans and pets. While a lot of commercial household cleaners are petroleum-based and contributes to the further depletion of our natural resources, baking soda is environmentally friendly and the safest choice to conventional cleaning products in the market. As a matter of fact, it is incomparable to the highly scented commercial products that are usually filled with unpronounceable chemical ingredients that are dangerous to health.

Baking Soda is the perfect all-purpose cleaner for the home. It dissolves dirt in water, cuts grease and lifts oils and discoloration with ease. It also lifts up buildup on scalps from conditioners, hairsprays, and other products. It is a food-safe cleaner that can safely be used to clean every surface in the home. With a little water added to it, it can be made into a paste or used dry. It does a great job of scouring pots, pans, ovens, stovetops among others.

As a deodorizing agent, it neutralizes all kinds of odors. Causative agents of the unpleasant odors such as strong acids from spoiled milk or strong bases from spoilt fish are effectively neutralized. Baking soda brings the acidic and basic odor molecules into an odor-free and neutral state, thus acting as a deodorizer. Baking soda also deodorizes when dissolved in water and can be used as a mouthwash to deodorize bad breathe or on plastic food containers to deodorize absorbed pickle smells.

Baking soda acts as a buffer. It helps to maintain a stable acid-alkali balance or pH (power of hydrogen) balance. This keeps the substance neither too alkaline nor too acidic.

Water is neutral with a pH of 7, acids have a pH that is less than 7 while alkaline solutions have a pH that is higher than 7. When baking soda comes in contact with an acidic or alkaline substance, it naturally neutralizes that pH.

Baking soda can cause acid solutions to become more basic and basic solutions to become more acid. Thus, it helps in balancing the acid in our body by neutralizing the stomach acid to relieve us of acid indigestion, sour stomach and heartburn. It also works the same way on irritated skin by soothing inflammation and relieving itches and pain.

It is advisable to use a brand of baking soda that is aluminum- free. This is not difficult to find as most of them are. However, there are still quite a few that may be contaminated with aluminum so it is better to be 100 percent sure and safe. Baking soda is a wonder and a quick solution to numerous household issues.

Why Use Baking Soda

Below are a few reasons you should use baking soda instead of the conventional cleaning products. Once you go through these information, you will definitely do away with chemical household cleaners once and for all!

It Is Toxic-Free

Nowadays, many store-bought cleaning products contain a lot of harmful toxins. It is dangerous to inhale or use these products. Harmful chemicals that may be contained in them include ammonia, perchloroethylene, chlorine and phthalates. Excessive use of these chemicals may cause cancer and lung damage.

Other ways chemicals in conventional cleaners may endanger human health include:

- Damaging the kidney and liver

- Causing chemical burns in the sinuses and esophagus.

- Damaging organs from skin exposure.

- Damaging the skin from prolonged exposure.

- Causing throat irritation.

- Swelling of the mouth and throat.

- Headaches and dizziness

It is Safe For Kids

Isn't it a great relief that you no longer need to be unduly worried about your kids stumbling on chemical cleaners or wondering whether you have kept the cabinets unlocked or left any chemicals out of the reach of an inquisitive child?

While you still need to lock up your non-toxic cleaning products in cabinets with child-proof locks, you are now less likely to worry about causing your children major health damage even if they come in contact with them.

Now not only are you worry-free but your kids can also follow you around, watch and even offer to help while you clean. It is also a great opportunity for you to teach them how to scrub the bathroom counters as they watch and imitate your move with a sponge.

... And Pets Too

Pets are at risk of inhaling and even directly ingesting toxic cleaning products. With their noses so close to the ground, they will sniff, lick and lay in spilled toxic cleaners. In the long run, these animals will suffer numerous health problems. You ought to protect these animals by switching to natural cleaners and keep them perpetually healthy.

Breathe Clean Air

Store-bought household cleaners being full of toxic chemicals pollute the air. After all, don't most of them come with warning labels about not directly breathing in the fumes? Sadly however, it is inhaled indirectly because they tend to linger in the air for a while. Furthermore, research has proven that the air quality inside a lot of homes can be two times to five times more contaminated than the air outside our homes. And this is caused by the household cleaners we use from day to day.

…And Drink Clean Water

Traditional cleaners seep into our water. The thing is, once you use them to clean, the volatile chemicals they contain get into the greater water cycle. While water treatment plants help to purify most of this water, it is difficult for them to effectively treat a large volume of these chemicals. Eventually, they find their way back to the water you use in your home.

So you see, you may be unknowingly contributing to a poisoned water supply. This is another reason you should go green so you do not add toxins and poisons back into the environment that produces the water.

Save Money- It's Good For Your Pocket

Most natural cleaning recipes are inexpensive. Baking soda, for instance is amazingly cheap it's almost a steal! They are even cheaper when bought in bulk. When compared to their synthetic counterparts, you get to save some good money at the end of every month.

They are easy to make as well, they will not take you much time, put one or two ingredients together and viola, you are good to go. The ingredients are readily available in grocery stores.

Get The Job Done- Naturally

Natural cleaners work! They have been tested and proven several times to be just as effective as synthetic cleaning products. It makes a lot of sense to switch as it still gets the job done.

KITCHEN CLEANING WITH BAKING SODA

Food Safe/Surface Safe kitchen
Why use harsh chemicals on your sinks, dish strainers and counters when dinner will still be made on those same surfaces?!

Simply sprinkle Baking Soda on a damp cloth, wipe clean, rinse thoroughly and dry.

You can also use this on cutting boards to eliminate onion smells and odors from previous cooking, backsplashes, plastic containers, microwaves, range hoods, oven tops and more!

By using this simple cleaning method, your kitchen will be clean and fresh.

Cleaning Coffee and Tea Pots:
Remove coffee and tea stains and get rid of bitter off-tastes by combining these 2 ingredients:

1/4 cup Baking Soda

1 quart warm water

For stubborn stains, add a little detergent in the solution soak overnight.

Remove unsightly stains from mugs and cups by scrubbing with sponge sprinkled with baking soda.

Deodorizing Dishwashers
Not ready to wash the dishes yet?

Sprinkle some Baking Soda in the bottom of the dishwasher or directly on the dishes to absorb the odors from the dishes. The baking soda does 2 things:

1. Deodorizes before the dishwasher is run and

2. Cleaning in the first wash cycle.

Easier Dish Washing

Bolster your liquid's detergent's cleaning power. Add 2 tablespoons of baking soda to the dish water or sink along with the detergent. This will help to cut food and grease on pots, pans and dishes.

Control dishwasher odors by simply sprinkling a little baking soda on the bottom of the dishwasher between loads.

Drains and Garbage Disposals

Deodorize drains and disposal by pouring Baking Soda down your drain while running warm tap water. The Baking Soda works by neutralizing acid and basic odors so you could have a fresh drain.

For your slow drains, pour about 1 cup soda down the drain, pour about 1/2 cup of salt and then pour boiling water over it. Drain should now run well with no nasty smell.

Sprinkle Baking Soda in garbage cans to minimize the smell. Sprinkle between layers of garbage as they accumulate.

You should also wash and deodorize garbage cans occasionally by making a solution of 1 cup of Baking Soda for every 1 gallon of water.

Fruit and Vegetable Scrub
Clean off residue and dirt on fresh fruit and vegetables. Sprinkle baking soda on a damp sponge, scrub and rinse. It's safe! Enjoy your fruits and veggies.

Pots & Pans Care
Thanks to Baking Soda, no more heavy scrubbing of pots and pans! Simply combine baking soda, hot water and dish detergent and pour on pots and pans. Let it sit for 10 minutes and then wash.

Alternatively, sprinkle baking soda on roasting pans and crusted casseroles and let sit for five minutes. Scrub and rinse gently.

Soften burnt-on food by sprinkling a generous amount of baking soda over pots and pans' surfaces. Add hot water and leave to soak for 10 minutes. Add baking soda to damp sponge and scrub.

Microwave Cleaning

Clean and deodorize your microwave. Add 4 tablespoons of Baking Soda to 1 quart water. Use this solution and then rinse with clear water.

Refrigerators

Baking soda works for exterior and interior cleaning of your refrigerator.

Dissolve 2 tablespoons of baking soda in 1 quart warm water. Wipe all surfaces.

For stubborn areas, use baking soda and water paste to clean.

Deodorize your refrigerator: open a box of baking soda and place inside. Replace after three months.

Kitchen Sink& Sponges

Clean your kitchen sink by sprinkling baking soda into it and add a little vinegar. Once it starts to bubble, scrub the sink with a brush and rinse.

Soak stale-smelling sponges in a strong baking Soda solution to keep them fresh.

Deodorizing Containers

Baking soda can keep your plastic food containers and thermos smelling fresh.

Sprinkle baking soda on damp sponge and wash items or add 2 tbsp baking soda to container, fill it with hot water, cover and shake well.

For strong odors, prepare a solution of 4 tbsp Baking Soda and 1 quart of warm water. Soak items in it. You will be amazed at the outcome!

Silverware Shiner/ Homemade Ash Metal Polish

Add equal parts baking soda and equal parts warm water together to make paste. Using a sponge, apply to silver. Rub, rinse, and buff dry.

To make a metal ash polish, combine 4 tablespoons baking soda and 2 cups wood ashes from a woodstove or fireplace. Add just enough water to make a paste. Dampen a sponge and use it to rub the mixture onto stainless steel, chrome, gold or silver plating. Rinse and dry.

Extinguishing Minor Fires

Use Baking soda to smother small flames in the kitchen. It works because heated baking soda gives off carbon dioxide, which helps to smother grease and electrical fires.

For small cooking fires from ovens, burners, fry-pans, broilers and grills, turn off electricity or gas (if you can do so safely). Stand back and toss handfuls of baking Soda at the base of the flame to put the fire out.

For small electrical fires from heaters, outlets and small appliances, unplug appliances if you can do so safely. Then stand back and toss handfuls of baking Soda at the base of the flame to put the fire out.

In both instances, call the fire department afterwards to ensure the fire is out. To avoid re- ignition, do not try to move the item until completely cooled. Never use water on electrical fires because it could lead to electrocution or shock. Never use Baking Soda in deep fat fryers so it does not splatter.

BATHROOM CLEANING WITH BAKING SODA

Bathroom Floor Cleaner
Baking Soda dissolves the grime and dirt from a bathroom tile or no-wax floor easily and quickly.

Add 1/2 cup Baking Soda to a bucket of warm water, mixing well.

Mop floor or tile and rinse clean. Let your floor sparkle.

Shiny Tiles & Sinks
Sprinkle a little Baking Soda on a damp sponge. Scrub sink, tile and tub as usual. Rinse well and wipe dry.

Homemade Bathroom Scrub
Mix ¼ cup of baking soda and 1 tablespoon of liquid detergent together. Add a little vinegar to make it thick and creamy. Use as needed.

Toothbrush Soak

Add ¼ cup baking soda to ¼ cup water, mixing thoroughly. Soak toothbrushes in mixture and let them stand overnight for a good cleaning.

Shower Curtains & Toilet bowl

To deodorize and clean your shower curtain, sprinkle Baking Soda on a damp brush. Scrub shower curtain, rinse clean and hang it up to dry.

To clean the toilet bowl, toss 1/2 cup of baking soda into it and scour with toilet brush.

Grout & Tile Stains Remover

Add 3 parts baking soda to 1part water to make paste. Apply to grout with toothbrush or with damp sponge.

Hard bathwater Softener

Add 1/2 cup of baking soda to your bath water and enjoy a relaxing and deodorizing soak

Septic Care:

Help your Septic System flow freely by treat the septic tank with baking soda.

Flush 1 cup of Baking Soda down the toilet every week to help maintain a good pH in your septic tank.

LAUNDRY WITH BAKING SODA

Your laundry room can do with baking soda. Here are ways to go about it:

Freshen Laundry Hampers

Keep the clothes hamper fresh until ready to wash by sprinkling a generous amount of baking soda between clothes layers. This also softens the clothes at wash time.

During washing, add 1/2 cup Baking Soda with your favorite detergent to freshen laundry and help liquid detergents work harder!

Stubborn Smell Remover

Remove stubborn and sour smells from clothes such as perspiration odors, musty smells from storage and sour towels used in the summer by adding 1/2 cup of Baking Soda to the rinse cycle. Your clothes will emerge clean and smelling fresh.

Alternatively, you can treat smelly clothes before wash time by soaking them for at least an hour in a solution of 1/2 cup baking soda and 1 gallon of warm water.

Chlorine Bleach Booster

Baking Soda will help your liquid chlorine bleach to work harder. Your whites will be whiter and fresher. Just add 1/2 cup Baking Soda to your usual amount of liquid bleach. For front loaders, add 1/4 cup.

Excellent Baby Laundry

Spits-up occur often. When it does, rub baking soda over bibs to cut odors and make laundry easier. To freshen cloth diapers, soak in a solution of 1/2 cup baking soda and 2 quarts of water. To clean and deodorize diaper pail, combine baking soda and water then use it to wipe the inside and outside of the pail.

Homemade Fabric Softener

Combine 1 cup baking soda, 6 cups distilled white vinegar and 8 cups water. This makes about a gallon and you can use 1 cup per regular load of laundry in the last rinse cycle.

Freshen Closets

Place a box of baking soda on the closet shelf to keep clothes smelling fresh.

PETS, TOYS AND PESTS

Porcupine Quill Remover
Add 2 teaspoons baking soda to 1 cup vinegar and apply to quill area.

After 10 minutes, reapply and wait again for 10 minutes. Quills should come from your pets easily.

Fido Dry-Cleaner
Baking soda is non-toxic and therefore safe to use around dogs. Rub a handful of baking soda into dog's fur and then comb it out. Dog will be clean and deodorized even without a bath. To brush your pets' teeth, add baking soda to toothbrush and use.

Toys And Dishes Cleaner

Soak your pet's dishes and toys in a solution of 3 tbsp baking soda and1 quart warm water. Keep pests away from your Fido's food bowls by surrounding bowl with baking soda.

Pet Bedding & Cages

Sprinkle baking soda over dry surface. Let it sit for 15 minutes, then vacuum. To clean small animal cage, sprinkle baking soda on damp sponge and wipe surfaces. Rinse and dry.

Fresh Kitty Litter

Spread baking soda on the bottom of kitty box. Cover with litter to maximize smells. Alternatively, make a litter by adding a small box of baking soda to 3 inches of sandy clay, mixing thoroughly.

Roaches And Silverfish Killer

Mix equal parts baking soda and sugar together. Place in an infected area. Bugs like sugar and will be drawn to them and end up eating too much baking soda which will kill them.

Keep Ants At Bay

Combine equal parts of baking soda and water. sprinkle mixture where there are ants.

Toys &Stuffed Animal Freshener

Keep cuddly stuffed animals fresh by sprinkling baking soda on them and leaving for 15 minutes. Simply brush off afterwards.

Clean other toys by using 1/4 cup baking soda and 1 quart warm water. Submerge these toys in this mixture and then rinse with clear water. You can also dampen a cloth with this mixture and wipe toys.

HYGIENE AND BEAUTY USES WITH BAKING SODA

Mouthwash/Bad Breath Killer

Make a mouthwash with baking soda by adding 1teaspoon of it to 1/2 glass of water. Swish through teeth and rinse. For those who suffer from bad breath, this solution is highly effective as baking soda does more just covering up the smell cause by bacteria but neutralizes it.

If you prefer a slightly more effective mouthwash that can kill bacteria and prevent gum disease and infection, add a pinch of salt to the solution. This is because salt (sodium) is disinfectant and kills off germs.

Homemade Toothpaste

Baking Soda is a mild dentifrice that helps to keep teeth white and clean.

To brush your teeth the natural way, add a little baking soda on a wet toothbrush and brush as usual. This will clean teeth and neutralize bacterial waste.

Dentures/ Retainers Freshener

Soak dentures, retainers, mouthpieces and other oral appliance in 2 teaspoons of Baking Soda and a small bowl of warm water. The Baking Soda works by loosening food particles and neutralizing odors to keep dentures or retainers fresh.

Refreshing Bath Additive

Have a refreshing bath. Add 1/2 cup of Baking Soda to your tub of water. The Baking Soda works by neutralizing acids on the skin and washing away oil and perspiration. Relax, enjoy your bath and emerge with skin that feels silky soft.

De-product Hair

When your favorite shampoo or conditioner no longer works on your hair, the likely cause is product build-up on your hair. Say goodbye to build-ups from mousses, sprays and conditioners with the help of baking soda.

Simply add1 teaspoon of Baking Soda to your regular shampoo bottle and wash hair. This will give you a natural clean hair and prevent product build ups well.

Alternatively, after shampooing hair, dissolve teaspoon baking soda in 1 cup of water or apple cider vinegar. Pour this mixture over your hair and rinse off with fresh, clean water.

Dry shampoo

To remove excess oils in your hair, dust hair with dry baking soda. This helps when you do not feel like shampooing. Use as a dry shampoo.

Hand Cleanser

Neutralize odors on hands and scour away ground-in dirt with a paste of 3 parts Baking soda added to 1 part water. Alternately use 3 parts Baking Soda added to 1 part liquid hand soap. Scrub and then rinse clean.

Nails Cleanser

Yellowing, stained nails are unsightly and can make your hands look older. Make a paste of equal parts baking soda and hydrogen peroxide. Afterwards, use a nail scrub brush to scrub on top of your nails and under it. Leave to sit for about 5 minutes and then rinse off. However, if your nails are persistently yellow, consult a doctor as this could be a sign of a fungal infection.

All- Natural Facial Scrub

Baking Soda can be used as an invigorating and gentle, facial scrub. Simply make a baking soda paste of 3 parts to 1 part water. Wash face with soap and water and then apply in a gentle circular motion. Rinse clean.

Soothing Foot Soak

Are your feet tired? Soak them for 10 minutes in a solution of 4 tbsp baking soda and 1 qt. warm water. It also provides relief from itchiness caused by athlete's foot and helps to soften calluses.

Natural Deodorant

Searching for a natural alternative to sticks and sprays? A pinch baking soda sprinkled under your arms will do. Alternatively, you may make a paste by mixing with water and if you cannot make it stick, add a little cornstarch to it.

To deodorize your shoes, simple sprinkle some baking soda in them. Baking soda also helps to minimize razor burns before and after shaving. Just add 1 tablespoon baking soda to 1 cup of water and apply to face.

Grooming Accessories Cleaner
Soak combs, brushes, cosmetic sponges, curlers and applicators overnight in a solution of 4 tablespoons baking soda and 1 quart of water. Rinse and leave to dry. This helps to clean hair product residue and natural oil build-up from such accessories like combs and brushes.

Silver Jewelry Polisher
Does your silver jewelry look old and tarnished? Try this recipe.

Pour very hot water into a small bowl and dip your jewelry in it. Now add 1 tablespoon of baking soda and 1 sheet of aluminum foil in the water. By doing this, the tarnish from your jewelry is transferred to the aluminum. Using a wooden device, move the pieces around, ensuring that the jewelry touches the aluminum. After a few minutes, rinse jewelry and polish with a soft cloth. Do not use this on organic material like pearls or jewelry with gemstones to avoid damage.

PERSONAL HEALTH CARE WITH BAKING SODA

Soothe minor burns and rashes

Make a paste by combining 3parts baking soda, 1 part witch hazel or water and apply. Recipe can be used for poison ivy itch as well.

Baking soda also helps to clear acne. Simply make a paste and spread it over your face. It works like magic!

Antacid Drug

Dissolve 1/2 teaspoon of baking soda in 1/2 glass of water. Drink slowly.

Insect Bite Care:

Make a Baking Soda paste and ease the pain and itching cause by an insect bite.

1. Remove the stinger.

2. Combine 3 parts Baking Soda to 1 part water and apply to the area affected.

3. Leave to dry, wash off and repeat if necessary.

Soothe Irritated Skin
Baking Soda helps to soothe the sting of minor burns, sunburn and windburn.

Make a baking soda solution of 4 tablespoons in 1 quart of water. Immerse a washcloth in the solution and apply to the affected area.

Alternatively, make a paste with 3 parts Baking Soda and 1 part water and then apply to the area.

Soothing Skin Bath
Add 1/2 cup Baking Soda to a bath of water. Enjoy your bath and be relieved of the itchy skin of poison ivy or prickly heat.

For localized rashes and irritations, make a paste using 3 parts Baking Soda and 1 part water.

Treat diaper rash by putting 2 tablespoons of bathing soda in your baby's bathwater.

Sore Throat Eliminator

Ease your sore throat by making a solution of baking soda and water and gargling every 4 hours. This works because baking soda eliminates the acids causing the pain.

Stuffy Nose

Add 1teaspoon of baking soda to your vaporizer. This will unblock your stuffy nose fast!

Neutralize Gassy Beans

Prevent gassy issue and aid digestion. Soak your beans as usual then sprinkle 1teaspoon of baking soda in the water.

AROUND THE HOME WITH BAKING SODA

Scuff Marks Remover/ Safer Front Steps

Remove scuff marks on your no-wax floor. Sprinkle Baking Soda on damp sponge, rub clean and then rinse. Baking Soda removes scuff marks without scratching the floor!

Skid-proof front steps by sprinkling baking soda liberally on icy steps and walkways.

Musty Books Deodorizer

Dry the books out then sprinkle a little baking soda between pages. Let it stay for 5 to 7 days then brush out.

Cleaner Walls & Carpets

Crayon marks from walls can be gently removed with baking soda. Rub with a damp sponge or cloth sprinkled with baking soda.

Deodorize your carpets. Sprinkle a lot of baking soda on carpets then leave for 15 minutes. Go ahead and vacuum.

Deodorize Smoke-Filled Room
Eliminate the haze and odor from your room by adding 1quart of warm water and 4tablespoons baking soda to a plant mister. Spray into the smoky air.

Fresher& Longer Lasting Flowers
Your cut flowers can be fresher and made to last longer with baking soda. Just add 1teaspoon of it to the water in the vase and that's it.

Make An Inexpensive Plaster
To make a plaster, make a paste by combining white glue and baking soda. Apply to cracks with a finger.

Shoes, Rubber Gloves & Chairs

To polish white baby shoes, sprinkle baking soda on them and rub with a damp sponge. Rinse shoes and buff.

Sweeten smelly sneakers by just sprinkling a little baking soda inside. Shake out before wearing.

If you are finding it hard to slip into your rubbers gloves after trying repeatedly, simply rub some baking soda into the fingers then you will be able to slip them on easily.

Clean your baby's high chair by using a solution of 4 tablespoons of baking soda in 1 quart of warm water. For really stained or very dirty ones, scrub directly with baking soda on a damp sponge.

Air Freshener

Mix baking soda with any perfumed bath salts that you choose. Transfer the mixture into small sachet bags and place indoors. The air will be freshened.

CARS AND GARAGES

Batteries Cleaner

Baking Soda is a mild alkali. Therefore, it can help to neutralize battery acid corrosion on cars. Begin by disconnecting the battery terminals then add 3parts Baking Soda and 1 part water together to form a paste.

Dampen a cloth and use to scrub corroded battery terminal. Re-connect the terminals once done then coat with petroleum jelly so corrosion does not occur again. A word of caution: batteries contain strong acid so be careful when working around them.

Cleaner Cars

Clean your car lights, windows, chrome, vinyl seats, tires and floor mats with baking soda.

Add Baking Soda to 1 quart warm water and apply this solution with a soft cloth or sponge to remove tree sap, road grime, tar and bugs.

For stubborn stains, sprinkle baking Soda onto a damp sponge and use. Rinse and then dry with a soft towel. The result is a clean and toxic-free car with streak-free windshield, freshened floor mats and brightened headlights.

Oil and Grease Stains Remover
Clean up grease spills and light-duty oil in your driveway or garage floor. Just sprinkle Baking soda directly on the spot and use a wet brush to scrub.

Cars Deodorizers
Eliminate odors from upholstery and carpets. Sprinkle baking Soda directly on them. Wait for at least 15 minutes and then vacuum.

Deodorize Car Ashtrays
To eliminate stale tobacco odors, just pour 1/2 inch of Baking Soda in the ashtray. It will

also help in extinguishing cigarettes and cigars. Replace Baking Soda weekly and empty ashtrays regularly.

RV Water Tanks Deodorizer

Protect your RV against rancid taste and sweeten it. Fill reservoir with 1 cup of baking soda dissolved in 1 gallon of warm water. Drain and flush then fill tank with plain water. Drain again and fill again with plain water. This works because the baking soda eliminates stale odors as well as the mineral buildup that leads to it.

BAKING SODA FOR OUTDOOR USE

Cleaning Grills

Clean up grill for the next barbecue. Sprinkle a little dry baking soda on a damp brush, scrub gently and rinse clean. Baking Soda won't scratch shiny surfaces and it cleans exterior surfaces such as trays and knobs very well.

Pool Care

Maintain a balanced swimming pool pH. The right pH protects the walls of your pools, its metal fittings and makes swimming in the water delightful instead of an itchy and unpleasant experience. A pH of 7.4 to 7.8 is the appropriate range for a swimming pool. However, if the pH of your pool registers as low after testing it, you can use baking soda to slightly raise your pH but do not to add too much baking soda because it is harder to lower total alkalinity than it is to raise it.

Baking soda's main task is to raise the total alkalinity of a pool. If the pH in your pool keeps dropping even after trying to raise it, test your total alkalinity. Total alkalinity should be between 80 ppm to 150 ppm. With low total alkalinity, the pH will fluctuates at random. If your test indicates a low total alkalinity, add 1.4 lbs of baking soda per 10,000 gallons of water in your swimming pool. This should increase the total alkalinity by at least10 ppm. Allow the water circulate for 1- 2 hours before testing again.

Cleaner Pool Tools

Clean plastic and vinyl pool toys and eliminates any mildew-like odors. Make a solution of 1/4 cup Baking Soda and1 quart warm water. Wipe down and rinse. For very dirty toys, dampen a sponge, sprinkle some baking Soda on it, scrub item and rinse.

Non-Toxic Homemade Fungicide

Add 4 teaspoons baking soda to 1 gallon of water. Spray on vines and grapes at the appearance of the first fruits. Spray once in a week for 2 months, and after each rain. It can also be sprayed on rosebushes to fight black spot fungus.

Rejuvenate The Greenery

Add 1 teaspoon of baking soda, 1 teaspoon of Epsom salt, 1/2 teaspoon of clear ammonia together in a gallon of water. For each rosebush-size shrub, use about1 quart of this solution and watch it regain its luster after a while.

Your beloved veggies are susceptible to consumption by rabbits. To prevent this from happening, spread baking soda around your flowerbeds.

You can also sweeten your tomatoes by sprinkling some baking soda around your tomato plants.

Power Cleaner

Spruce up your fishing gear by making baking soda solution and then using it to clean rods, hooks, lines and buckets. There's no need to worry as baking soda will not pollute rivers and lakes. Cleanse your hands from gardening grime by rubbing baking soda on wet hands and rinsing afterwards.

Clean Lawn Furniture

Add 1/4 cup of Baking Soda to 1 quart of warm water. Use this solution to clean and deodorize patio and pool furniture. Rinse clean.

For tougher stains, sprinkle the baking Soda directly on a damp cloth or sponge, scrub and rinse.